PRE 1949
ACUPUNCTURE

PRE 1949
ACUPUNCTURE

Andrew Mcpherson

Library of Congress Control Number: 2019910344
ISBN: Hardcover   978-1-7960-0483-0
               Softcover   978-1-7960-0482-3
               eBook   978-1-7960-0484-7

Print information available on the last page.

Rev. date: 04/14/2023

To order additional copies of this book, contact:
Xlibris
AU TFN: 1 800 844 927 (Toll Free inside Australia)
AU Local: (02) 8310 8187 (+61 2 8310 8187 from outside Australia)
www.Xlibris.com.au
Orders@Xlibris.com.au
794725

CONTENTS

PREFACE

I am presenting this book as an introduction to the subject matter of pre-1949 acupuncture and Chinese medicine. While much of what I have to say may be controversial to some, there is no denying the research behind this topic. In addition, I hope that, overall, this book will help the seasoned practitioner, the lay person, and the aspiring student alike, to clarify matters rather than ultimately confuse them.

Finally, I would like to thank my wife, my friends, and my students for their much- needed help in getting this book published. Without their assistance, none of this would have been possible.

Andrew McPherson

INTRODUCTION

Where to begin?

When we talk about traditional Chinese medicine (TCM), we are actually referring to something we consider to be Chinese obviously. But insofar as one of its major components, acupuncture, is concerned, nothing could be farther from the truth, as this book will show.

It is true, that the Japanese, and understandably the Koreans, Thai, Vietnamese, etc., have developed acupuncture along their own lines and have their own theories along the way. However, what we will be referring to would be so much more than that.

When we discuss acupuncture, we are referring to an area which the Chinese consider to be 5,000–6,000 years old; and which people often refer to as *The Huang di Nei Jing* (*The Yellow Emperor's Classic of Internal Medicine*), the first medical book ever written in the history of man. While, on the other hand, many Western scholars seem to take great delight in belittling acupuncture and saying it is 2,000 or 3,000 years old, at best.

In actual fact, these two ideas may not be the case at all. Acupuncture, may be really much older. For the purpose of demonstrating this, I will ask the reader for some leeway on this matter and to reserve judgement till the end of my argument.

In order to understand much of the history of acupuncture, we may have to travel back to the anti-Diluvium times (i.e., before the Deluge). Many scientists and scholars now believe the Deluge or Great Flood did, in truth, exist but that it was 7,000 years ago not 3,000–4,000 years ago, if one believes the biblical scholars. Sediment dredged from the Black Sea shows that a real flood did engulf most of the then-known earth. With this in mind, we must realise that much of what we now call 'history' didn't begin until 7,000 years ago and maybe even before then.

This does not give us licence to say whatever we want. However, there are many things that don't make sense and tend to point to an earlier knowledge of acupuncture by a number of nations and not just China.

<u>Ancient cavemen and tattoos</u>

One first stop along the way in this amazing story begins in the fairly primitive and what some consider pretty basic times—a few years ago. Newspapers reported a group of people, the Otsi, who had been unearthed from ice in parts of Europe—Tyrol to be precise. Some of these people that were unearthed had tattoos on them, and researchers were quite perplexed by this until they realised what the tattoos were for. They were suddenly confronted by the conclusions–actually instructions from one acupuncturist to another—telling them that the certain points identified and marked (appearing as tattoos) were the best points to use to treat this particular individual.

It is not inconceivable that early man, maybe even via accident, had discovered acupuncture points. In fact, the Chinese have, for a number of decades, maintained that primitive man had discovered acupuncture/acupressure points by using sharp stones called 'bian'.

In addition, the Chinese have also maintained that later on, soldiers wounded by swords or arrows quite often got better, rather than worse, because these weapons had inadvertently stimulated acupuncture points.

What are the possibilities that those things had also happened in the West? How unlikely is it that they hadn't happened?

<u>Herbs and acupressure points in Africa</u>

During the 1990s, there were, and still are, many fads regarding acupuncture. One of these fads was particularly interesting and involved using herbal ointments and involved their use on acupressure points or zones. Just as was said in the newspaper articles, at the time, this had been done by native tribes in Africa for hundreds of years. These articles claimed that rather than using somewhat more painful Chinese acupuncture, the same or similar effect could be obtained by using these herbal ointments. While the practice didn't last long, it was very popular at the time.

Does this mean that African tribes knew something about acupuncture points? Although the previous example and this example doesn't show any great in-depth development of theoretical understanding normally shown in TCM or traditional Chinese medicine. However, these examples, if verified, indicate that acupuncture may have been around since before the *The Huang di Nei Jing* book. We know that much of the information contained in the *Nei Jing* is now considered by even the Chinese to have come from earlier works such as the *Yi jing*. In fact, there are many references made in the *Nei Jing* to experiences learnt from in prior times. If we refer once more to the anti-Diluvium world, acupuncture may really be Babylonian or earlier, or simply and understandably well known by many cultures. Therefore, the Chinese can be seen as the custodians of acupuncture or the 'keepers of the key' while also developing the system even if others have forgotten it.

<u>Foot reflexology and ancient peoples</u>

Foot reflexology, or zone therapy as it has become known, is not actually acupuncture, but most practitioners of both acupuncture and reflexology agree that it is based on the same principles. While only one acupuncture point really appears on the sole of the foot, there are many 'zones' which are linked to the main channels by branches. North American Indian tribes and certain African tribes not only knew about foot reflexology, but ancient Egyptian tombs dating back from 2370 BC had in them drawings of foot massage.

<u>Ancient Chinese writings</u>

When researching a number of ancient texts which purportedly quoted and exemplified even more ancient techniques, I personally have found many references to methods coming from 'countries overseas'. One's first reaction is to think of Japan, which has had a kind of off-again-on-again relationship with China for hundreds of years, but the references seemed to predate China's exchanges with Japan. So what are these mysterious 'other countries' who supplied China with information about acupuncture?

CHAPTER 1

The Pulse Classic

The problem seems to have been with book *The Pulse Classic* or *Mai jing* as it is popularly known. Representing a separation between old and new, the Mai jing is considered by most Chinese medicine doctors to be an abandonment of ancient practices, and their underlying diagnoses and treatment, in favour of the new.

Don't get me wrong, *The Pulse Classic* was, and still is, a great book. However, it has remained questionable considering its many additions and deletions or omissions, let alone the numerous versions (there are at least three) it has had—talk about 'throwing the baby out with the bath water'. What is more likely the case is that the author of *The Pulse Classic,* Wang Shu he, meant his book to be an addition or an updating of the knowledge of pulse diagnoses. Instead, we are faced with a substitution of old old views with a lot of new ideas which, like I said, have been altered and added to over time. (A not uncommon habit and often considered to be the case in the cases of even the *Su wen* and the *Ling shu.)*

In one particular section of *The Pulse Classic,* Wang Shu he when clarifying more about the san bu and the jiu hou (the three sections and the nine parts) system of pulse diagnosis, says that not only can a bowstring moderate pulse, for example, be a sign of the liver affecting the spleen, but that the actual relevant pulse positions can become affected (see below):

Figure 1

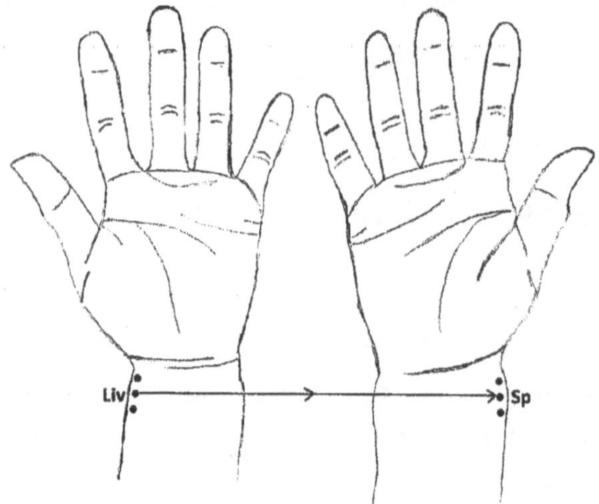

Well and good, but he goes on to say that over a period of time, it is difficult to see where problems really begin (see below).

Figure 2

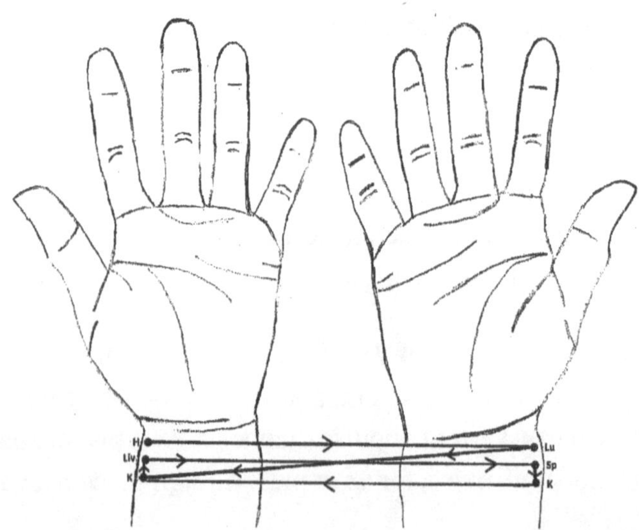

To the acupuncturist or Chinese herbal medicine practitioner, this can be a real problem; and I'm sure you can see why. Because this form of pulse-taking is seemingly devoid of time combinations, etc. as it leaves things open for too much interpretation insofar as the seasons and the years. Even the *Pi Wei Lun* (the treatise on spleen and stomach) by Li Dong yuan considered much of this.

In fact, there have been many questions over pulse positions for many centuries, and there is still no definitive decision regarding the matter (see table below).

Table 1. Cun Kou Diagnosis Methods Zang-Fu Methods Zang-Fu Clarification.

	CUN		GUAN		CHI		
	Left	Right	Left	Right	Left	Right	
Nei Jing	Heart Tan Zhong	Lung Chest Centre	Liver Diaphragm	Spleen Stomach	Kidney Abdomen	Kidney Abdomen	
Nan Jing	Heart Small intestine	Lungs Large intestine	Liver Gall bladder	Spleen Stomach	Kidney Urinary bladder	Kidney Ming Men	Large small intestines match heart lungs, Biao Li mutually belongs right kidney belongs fire, therefore ming men also hou at chi.
Mai Jing	Heart Small intestine	Lungs Large intestine	Liver Gall bladder	Spleen Stomach	Kidney Urinary bladder	Kidney Triple heater	
Jing Yue Chuan Shu	Pericardium Heart Luo	Lungs Tan Zhong	Liver Gall bladder	Spleen Stomach	Urinary bladder Kidney Large intestines	Triple heater Kidney Ming Men Small intestines	Large intestines match left chi is metal water mutually from small intestines match right chi is fire return to fire position.

Yi Zong Jin Pian	Heart Tan Zhong	Lungs chest centre	Liver Gall bladder Diaphragm	Spleen Stomach	Urinary bladder Kidney Large intestines	Kidney Large intestines	

While on the subject, Wang Shu he in *The Pulse Classic* favoured radial pulse diagnosis and treatment, whereas other earlier classics tend to support more 'body points' diagnosis, etc. And, in fact, many old, old classics talk about the radial pulse being 'not true' and the body pulses, on the other hand, as being 'true' (see the following table on parts diagnosis):

Table 2

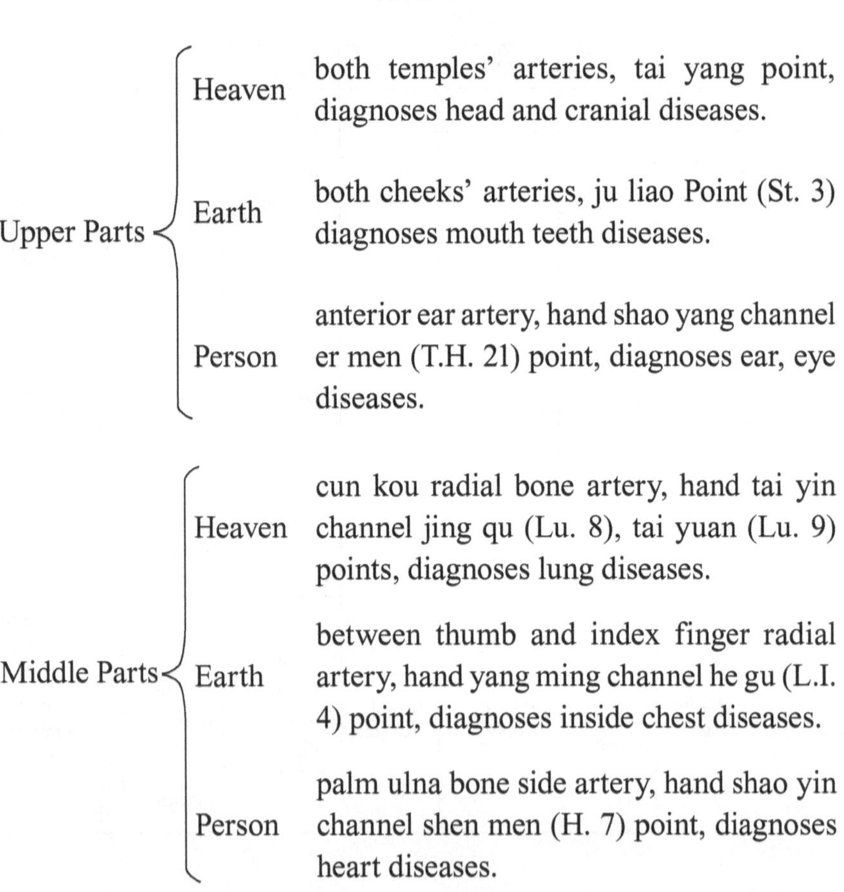

Upper Parts	Heaven	both temples' arteries, tai yang point, diagnoses head and cranial diseases.
	Earth	both cheeks' arteries, ju liao Point (St. 3) diagnoses mouth teeth diseases.
	Person	anterior ear artery, hand shao yang channel er men (T.H. 21) point, diagnoses ear, eye diseases.
Middle Parts	Heaven	cun kou radial bone artery, hand tai yin channel jing qu (Lu. 8), tai yuan (Lu. 9) points, diagnoses lung diseases.
	Earth	between thumb and index finger radial artery, hand yang ming channel he gu (L.I. 4) point, diagnoses inside chest diseases.
	Person	palm ulna bone side artery, hand shao yin channel shen men (H. 7) point, diagnoses heart diseases.

<table>
<tr><td rowspan="3">Lower Parts</td><td>Heaven</td><td>big thigh, internal side upper section, foot jue yin channel we li (Liv. 10) point, women select tai chong (Liv. 3) point diagnoses liver diseases.</td></tr>
<tr><td>Earth</td><td>internal ankle back heal bone artery, foot Shao yin channel tai xi (K. 3) point, diagnoses kidney diseases.</td></tr>
<tr><td>Person</td><td>big thigh, internal side upper section, foot tai yin channel ji men (Sp. 11) point. Hou stomach qi uses chong yang (St. 42) point, diagnoses spleen and stomach's diseases.</td></tr>
</table>

In addition, the Buddhists have their own system of pulse diagnosis. Remember, the Buddhists have had a lot of experience in martial arts as well as in medical arts. Long before there were any hospitals, the Buddhist monks were treating the general populace. According to the Buddhists, the pulses were very different at least as far as radial pulses (i.e., cun, guan, chi) are concerned (see below):

Table 3

Three parts	MEN				WOMEN			
	Left hand		Right hand		Left hand		Right hand	
	Chinese Medicine	Zang Medicine	Chinese Medicine	Zang Medicine	Chinese Medicine	Zang Medicine	Chinese Medicine	Zang Medicine
Cun	Heart Small intestine	Heart Small intestine	Lung Large intestine	Lung Large intestine	Heart Small intestine	Lung Large intestine	Lung Large intestine	Heart Small intestine
Guan	Liver Gall bladder	Spleen Stomach	Spleen Stomach	Liver Gall bladder	Liver Gall bladder	Spleen Stomach	Spleen Stomach	Liver Gall bladder
Chi	Kidney Urinary bladder	Left Kidney Triple heater	Mingmen Triple heater	Right Kidney Urinary bladder	Kidney Urinary bladder	Left Kidney Triple heater	Mingmen Triple heater	Right Kidney Urinary bladder

Zang medicine refers to medicine influenced by the Taoist and Buddhist scripture.

Finally, at least one of the Classics lists the pulses as moving, not static. In other words, *yin* and *yang* can change according to the year (see below):

And there is also the three parts (of the body) diagnosis (see the following table):

Table 4

Upper	Ren Ying (ST 9)	Throat artery	Stomach Qi
Middle	Cun Kou (Lu 9)	Radial artery	12 Channels and Zang Fu's Qi
Lower	Fu Yang (St 42)	Foot dorsal artery	Stomach Qi

Theoretical, you say. In reality, no. There are many acupuncture point prescriptions, and even more, herbal medicine prescriptions that are admittedly quite old, which look at diagnosing and treating the patients according to their body points.

For example, 'The fu yang mai floating and uneven, shao yin mai as if undertaken, various yin slow become attack of the viscera, its illness is at the spleen, a technique should be used to promote downward unblocking. How do you know this is true? If those who have a pulse floating big, qi excess blood deficient. The fu mai floating and uneven, stomach qi deficient. If the shao yin mai is bowstring and floating, it can be seen all becomes a "complete" pulse, so undertaken. If the opposite, slippery and rapid, so knows its pus.' (*Shan han jin gui wen ging ming zhu ji chen*, book 1, p.18.)

Furthermore, 'The urinary bladder rules heaven, cold atmosphere suo triumphs, then cold qi adversely arrives, blood changes at the inside, and as a result occurs ulcers, and people have jue heart pain, vomiting blood, diarrhoea with blood, nose bleeding, tendency to be unhappy, sometimes dizzy collapses, if yun fire blandly, sudden rain moreover sodden, the chest and abdomen are stuffy, hands hot, elbows spasmed, armpits swelling, heart has big palpitations, chest ribs and gastric cavity not peaceful, face red eyes yellow, tendency to burp, dry throat, in extreme cases then colour ashen, thirsty and likes drinks, or illness at the heart. Shen men (H7) jue (dies), dies and can't treat (difficult to treat).' (*Huang di nei jing su wen yun qi qi pian jian jie*, p. 706).

Figure 3

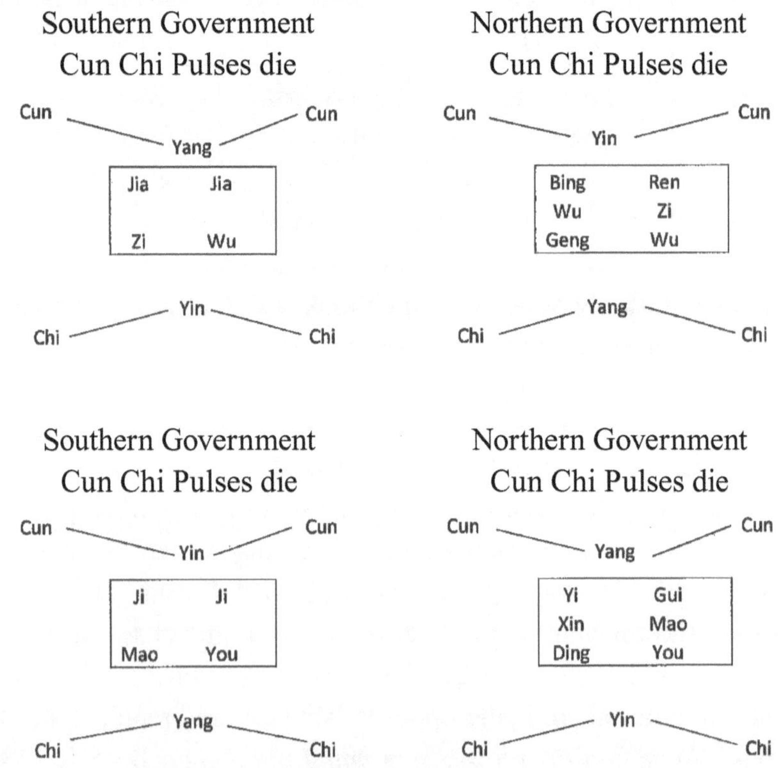

All these show that rather than pulse diagnosis being universally standardised (or uniform) as we've been told, there are many theories, none completely agreed upon or generally accepted. Pulse diagnosis, as we've seen, tends to be a result of and dictator of acupuncture and Chinese herbal medicine prescription and the TCM theory. If modern Chinese medicine ignores all this and pretends everything is standardised even after thousands of years of indecision, maybe we're seeing the Chinese 'turning a blind eye' to so much, including other approaches to diagnosing and treating people, thereby along the line of their more recent conclusions, which may be dictated by politics and a desire to provide modern-day students with a more simple, 'user-friendly' system.

CHAPTER 2

Pre-1949 and post-1949 Acupuncture and Traditional Chinese Medicine

Whether accidental or not, there were obviously problems with acupuncture and TCM before 1949. What happened after 1949 is nothing short of incredible, if not, in many ways, downright disastrous.

To give things their true context, maybe we should remember when the communists took over China in 1949, China was a society that was largely uneducated (i.e., very few people could read or write), largely underfed and undernourished (i.e., many people were starving), and rife with corruption (which led to the economy and Chinese society stagnating for a lot of decades). First and foremost, the Chinese needed a lot of doctors, regardless of whether they were adept at Chinese medicine or Western medicine. Initial attempts to bring in practitioners, who were called Barefoot doctors, ended in disaster. For many reasons, this idea failed, partly because these Barefoot doctors were poorly trained (on the average, they were lucky to have a year's training), and partly because they were unable to meet the needs of the people (i.e., they chased after nomadic tribes which had by then moved on).

These early attempts told the Communist government that any chance to teach proper and genuine acupuncture and TCM to the Chinese people just wasn't going to work. The initial doctors who advocated a return to traditional Chinese acupuncture, like Professor Chen Dan an, were only listened to in part. The Chinese government could undoubtedly see that the reestablishment of real acupuncture and TCM would take years, maybe even decades. To a certain extent, the Chinese government listened to Chen Dan an but to a greater extent they listened to their committees—something communism is noted for (i.e., the word Soviet means 'committee').

To add fuel to the fire, Chinese Communism was, in the '50s, '60s, and early '70s, going through a philosophical battle. The Cultural Revolution pretty much insisted that doctors come up with a new form of Communist acupuncture; different to the old but with a loose basis in tradition (e.g., see ear acupuncture).

By integrating some of the old with much of the new, the Chinese came up with a system that appealed to the scientific community and had a Western medicine basis to it. Because the main system was so Western medicine-orientated, it found support in those Chinese doctors who had already learnt a lot of Western medicine, plus it was easy to teach. And even better, this new system was marketable and could be taught to large number of practitioners overseas. This appealed to hardline Stalinist activists who wanted to see a furthering of 'the cause'. So overall, everyone was happy, or so it seemed.

The only thing that was yet to be addressed by all, given this somewhat political manouvring, was the main aim of acupuncture in the first place. The basic textbook for acupuncture for most colleges is *Chinese Acupuncture and Moxibustion* (Foreign Languages Press, Beijing) and has been so since the 1980s.

In the first chapter of this book, it actually states 'the ancient physicians had a preliminary understanding of pulse, blood, body fluid, qi, shen (manifestations of vitality), essence, five sounds, five colours, five flavours, six qi, eight winds, etc., as well as the ideology of relevant adaptation of the human body to natural environment.'

And then again later, 'Historically it derives from observations of the natural world made in early times by the Chinese people in the course of their lives and productive labour.' How many times have we been told that Chinese medicine is about man (person) and his/her environment. Despite this, the environment (heaven-tian, earth-di) is only paid lip service at the very least. For further examples of this, not only can one refer to the abovementioned textbook itself, but I would suggest the reader look at *The Chinese Way in Medicine* by Edward H. Hume.

<u>Further arguments</u>

Further evidence of this older system of Chinese medicine can be found in many of the terms of acupuncture: the 'ba feng' (eight winds), 'shi dong' and 'suo shen bing' (as explained by Professor Guan Zun hui in his book *On theory and clinical application of Channels and Collaterals*), 'to break channels' and 'broken channels', 'ying' and 'bu ying', 'tian' and 'di', and 'tian' and 'quan', etc.

While there are a vast number of terms that apply to acupuncture alone, there are also many terms which simply apply to Chinese herbal medicine. For example, 'those ying and duo (fall in with, add to the channel, that is, a little too much), calm and enable ('an de') without making deficiency (that is, make xu); those sui and ji (follow, all in the same boat, subtract from the channel that is, a little too little) calm and enable without making excess (that is, make shi)' *(Xue gu zhen ze,* 1991 p.147). This is an example, where there is no discernable 'xu' or 'shi'.

In Chinese herbalism, some herbs like dan shen *(Salvia multiorrhizae)* are the *red* equivalent to ginseng. However, they don't use the terms 'chi' or 'hong' as usual. Likewise, there is also a xuan shen *(Scrofularia ningpoensis),* sometimes called 'hei' shen, the *black* equivalent to ginseng. Again, no one uses the term 'hei' shen all that much, instead using 'xuan'. What, these two terms refer to is, in fact, the Chinese astrological view of things. In the Chinese view, 'dan' and 'xuan' refer to the identification of various stars and the consideration of what is a 'good' colour (*Shen mi de xing xiang* p.3, 2; *Huang di nei jing su wen yun qi qi pian jiang jie, Xue gu zhen ci*), unlike certain man-made reds and blacks. These 'natural' colours are, according to the Chinese, much easier to the eye and have many latent properties. At this point, one thinks of the old Catholic church idea of 'the doctrine of signatures'.

Following on from this, tastes and smells of herbs also play an important part in Chinese herbalism, not simply 'gui jing' (follow the channels), which has appealed to so many Westerners. Also, there are terms like 'thick' and 'thin', and 'heavy' and 'light', which have significant uses and applications (see Guan Zun hui's book *On the Theory and Clinical Application of Channels and Collaterals*).

Traditional Chinese acupuncture and herbal medicine have its own philosophy which undoubtedly conflicted with the Chinese Communists in the early days, so it was changed or disregarded. Likewise, many today would disagree with my conclusions in acupuncture and herbal medicine and say that various things are not scientific. But that really relates to your parameters and definition of 'science'. Once, people couldn't have conceived of man going to the moon or atomic submarines. Now, these things are reality.

CHAPTER 3

Acupuncture Today

My own clinical experience is that what has become known as modern standardised acupuncture can, at best, cure about 85 per cent of patients. I recently had a student under me, and he had studied with a doctor and an eminent naturopath. He said the doctor was able to cure about 50–55 per cent of patients and the naturopath, about 70 per cent, but he said that I was able to cure about 80–85 per cent of patients. Since then, I would say that this success rate has improved to almost 90 plus per cent. However, I wanted things to be even better. For a long time, I tried various things to improve my success rate further, but to no avail.

In the last few years, I have applied pre-1949 acupuncture and Chinese herbal medicine and have obtained great results. The problem with post-1949 acupuncture is that it is Western medicine-orientated. One of the old sayings in acupuncture and TCM is that 'bad doctors try to treat the disease, a good doctor treats the person, and very good doctors treat a nation.' (I am not so good a doctor as to treat a nation, but I have realised that chasing a disease is like a dog chasing its own tail). How many times have acupuncturists quoted this saying but don't actually listen to their own words. In other words, the idea is, and should be, to create balance in the body and the disease will go. But Westernized acupuncturists don't have enough faith so they cling to a symptomatic watered-down system of acupuncture. (Yes, we do have 'gui jing' or 'return to the channels' in Chinese herbal medicine and this is symptomatic in practice. And we do have something similar in acupuncture. Most of this is of secondary concern though and not of fundamental or primary concern.)

When it comes down to it, the Chinese Communists have 'watered-down' not only acupuncture and Chinese herbal medicine, but also tai-chi and even Chinese language. (When talking to an old Chinese woman recently, she commented on how when she went back to PRC China recently, people couldn't understand her when she talked about various things including festivals because these things no longer existed in the Chinese language). In effect, the Chinese performed a 'year zero' on the Chinese people; maybe not as bloody and violent as Cambodia but still as extensive. (There were also a lot of seemingly insurmountable problems, like I have already mentioned. Problems relating to basic education, food availability, and social issues, in general.)

In some ways, in the West, we see much of the same thing. But at the same time, don't get me wrong. If the more modernised system of acupuncture and TCM didn't exist, I doubt whether I would have gone on to practice Chinese medicine in the first place. To comprehend truly traditional concepts in TCM requires a big step in understanding. However, I do feel now would be a good time to rectify what I consider the mistakes of the past.

CHAPTER 4

Appropriateness of Points versus Point Indications

Describing the difference between pre-1949 and post-1949 acupuncture and TCM is a bit like describing rain to someone who has never seen it. Don't laugh. I have actually seen a case like this. Much of what is presented as post-1949 acupuncture is practised according to the use of point functions and indications. However, in pre-1949 acupuncture, point functions and indications have an almost secondary or tertiary level of importance, as already stated.

For example, I once used ST.25 on a patient in more recent times, not because of its functions and indications but because of what I call its 'appropriateness' or 'suitability'. ST.25 (tian shu) is normally used in post-1949 Chinese acupuncture for the following: abdomen pain, too much gas, abdominal distension, constipation and/or diarrhoea, weight loss, etc. But in pre-1949 acupuncture as well as being on the halfway mark body-wise, it has a special purpose. To go into this purpose would take an incredibly long time and wouldn't give this system its proper due. Needless to say, the patient had none of the usual indications called for (he had hemiplegia) when using this point, but it worked. In other words, people can be helped to get better without relying on functions and indications of points.

If one relies solely on functions and indications of points, isn't this really 'falling into the trap' of standardisation, which is already having disastrous effects on our medical systems. Additionally, isn't this relegating Chinese acupuncturists to the status of therapists, not unlike physiotherapists, occupational therapists, and even chiropractors. When really one should be regarding Chinese acupuncturists as doctors of a system or part of a system of medicine. In truth, in ancient times, Chinese practitioners used scalpels or scalpel-like instruments to treat people because acupuncture back then was part of the field of surgery or least 'wai ke' (external medicine). Having said that, so much can be achieved without the need for actual surgery, and Chinese acupuncture if practised properly is still a system of medicine. By using the pre-1949 system of acupuncture, I have found that the human body is remarkably resilient and, if not under the influence of a lot of superfluous drugs, has a tendency to get better by itself. One of the objects of traditional pre-1949 acupuncture is then to gently push or encourage the body (and mind) in the right direction—the right direction being better and better health.

Therefore, not only do we have 'zhi ben' (treat the underlying cause) as one of our overall basic precepts (as should be the case with any system or type or interpretation of acupuncture), but there are so many different variables, especially with pre-1949 acupuncture, making any comparison with physiotherapy, occupational therapy, or chiropractic, etc., positively remote. Finally, although inspection, auscultation, olfaction, and inquiry are extremely important for the practise of both pre-1949 and post-1949 acupuncture, palpation (feeling of the pulses) is more so for the proper use of pre-1949 acupuncture. However, new students to palpation initially may not need to rely on this as long as the other factors are taken into strict account.

CHAPTER 5

The Strange Case of Master Huang

Noted tai-chi master Master Huang Sheng xian, is the subject of this chapter. While it may seem strange to talk about a tai-chi master in a book that is discussing pre-1949 Chinese medicine, he is the perfect example of someone who truly understood traditional acupuncture but unfortunately was under-appreciated by both the tai-chi and Chinese medicine communities. Having read the Chinese language version of one of his two books, it is obvious that he had a very good grasp of pre-1949 TCM. In fact, when one reads his book, it is clear that his book is less about tai-chi and more about how it fits into Chinese 'cosmology' and an understanding of life. This is decidedly marred by ancient Chinese medical jargon and a sort of 'code' that is used in cases such as this.

Master Huang was considered a doctor of medicine at a village level. Nothing could be farther from the truth. After reading just a few pages of one of his books, one has no doubt that this was not really the case. (TCM doctors at village level were not party to the intricacies of TCM and were called 'practitioners of natural medicine' which does not describe Master Huang's knowledge of the subject.) More than likely, Master Huang was one of the many who was subject to and wanted to escape Communist rule and understated his qualifications or background to escape his circumstances.

From the very outset, one can see that Master Huang was not just talking about tai-chi but its place in TCM. Furthermore, he uses terms such as 'tian' (heaven) and 'di' (earth), etc., which are not used in everyday tai-chi, then or now. Writing about tai-chi in the scheme of things is nothing new. Since the twelfth century, this is quite popular amongst teachers and scholars of the art. And one could go further to say that many of the forms of tai-chi refer ultimately to the 'ba gua' (eight trigrams). In addition, noted modern-day practitioner Glenn Blythe often refers to 'open' and 'close', which is very similar to the Chinese medicine use of the terms 'kai' (open), 'he' (balance), and 'shu' (close). While the use of the form 'far lady uses the shuttle' is basically like the 'in-betweens' in Chinese medicine.

Of course, part of the problem is the *shoddy* translation that many of the old and new texts are subjected to. Combined with a misunderstanding about like I said, the Chinese 'cosmology' of things, no wonder so many concepts of tai-chi (and acupuncture) are not only undervalued but are inevitably even maligned. One such example is that of K1 (yong quan) which firstly wrongly called 'the bubbling well' when it is actually 'the gushing fountain'. (Not a big difference, I agree. But very big when you consider TCM concepts such as 'tian' and 'quan'.) In addition, many tai-chi practitioners now believe that the Chinese 'got it wrong' when viewing K1 as the point of balance of the human body. After having seen many of the ancient and modern classics on the subject, I can categorically say, 'This is not correct.' Nowhere in the ancient or modern texts do they actually mention 'point of balance', which is a Western medical term, possibly a physiotherapy one. What they do mention is that K1, not only is the main acupoint on the foot, but that it should touch the ground in order for it to connect with 'di' (earth). This hardly seems important, but from a TCM point of view, it is enormously important. Tai-chi is both a connection between heaven and earth. In reality, human beings are said to be the product of 'heaven and earth uniting'.

Obviously, what Master Huang was doing was trying to show his contemporaries that tai-chi was, in fact, a form of Chinese medicine. However, by the time Master Huang had published his books, acupuncture and TCM in general had significantly changed. Much of what he wrote was misunderstood and its context severely destroyed. Master Huang was simply another casualty in the war being waged by post-1949 acupuncture.

CHAPTER 6
Case Studies

<u>Case study 1</u>: Torticollis (Wry neck). Patient was a middle-aged woman who had a very bad chronic wry neck with extreme spasms. Both chiropractors and Western medicine doctors had given up on curing her. After half a dozen treatments, the neck pain disappeared and movement recovered. However, the shape of the trapezius muscle was still not normal, so three more treatments were given, and then her condition completely reverted to normal. Acupuncture and Chinese herbal medicine in keeping with the principles of pre-1949 TCM were given from the very start.

<u>Case study 2</u>: Hereditary high blood cholesterol. Even as a young girl, despite exercise and diet, patient had 7.8 cholesterol. When she came to the clinic, her cholesterol was over 8. (Her doctors even expressed concern about her having a heart attack). The problem was made much worse by the use of Western medicine for her breast cancer she had suffered from. After treatment for a couple of months of acupuncture and Chinese herbal medicine, along pre-1949 lines, the cholesterol was reduced to less than 4.1. The pulses also improved.

<u>Case study</u>: Acoustic neuromas. Patient was presented with acoustic neuromas. In other words, he had benign tumours in the ears and was losing his hearing, and so had to wear hearing aids. Doctors of Western medicine informed him there was no medicine for his

problem, and no operation could be performed on his ears. Out of desperation, the patient sought help from Chinese medicine. Pre-1949 acupuncture was given and Chinese herbal medicine was administered. The results were better than expected. Within three to four weeks, the patient reported that he not only felt good, but he quite often forgot to use his hearing aids.

Case study 3: Arthritis of the foot. Patient had suffered for a number of years from pains in the sides and dorsum of the foot. There had been no apparent injury to that foot. Pain quite often got very intense. Acupuncture plus moxa plus Chinese herbal medicine, in the form of pills, were applied. After two treatments, the pain was less intense and more intermittent. After three treatments, overall the pain was minimal but the patient lived very far away so it was impossible to see if she fully recovered.

Case study 4: Chronic neurosis. After exhibiting depressive behaviour and neurotic thinking for many decades, the patient was referred to the author for acupuncture and Chinese herbal medicine. The patient had problems sleeping and was at the verge of crying much of the time. After about half a dozen treatments, the patient declared, 'Is it possible to feel better than I have ever felt?!' From all the signs, the patient had decidedly improved.

Case study 5: Chronic hepatitis. According to Western medicine blood tests, the patient had hepatitis. He also complained about pain in the liver area. Aside from giving pre-1949 acupuncture and Chinese herbal medicine tablets, he received regular check-ups and blood tests from his doctor. The doctor reported actual improvement in his blood tests. Additionally, he felt better and had less liver pain. On the other hand, tests conducted on hepatitis patients in South Australia using standard acupuncture and Chinese herbal medicine failed to produce any real results. The patient we're discussing, continued to get better and better results.

<u>Case study 6</u>: Chronic depression. Patient was a man in his 60s. He not only suffered from insomnia but also was very unhappy about not being able to see his grandchild. In addition, he suffered from globus hystericus. Upon receiving pre-1949 acupuncture, his globus hystericus was greatly lessened, his insomnia got better, and his depression improved. This was all after only about a month's worth of treatments, at twice a week, and he didn't require any Chinese herbal medicine.

CHAPTER 7

Discovery

The discovery of what I have termed 'pre-1949' acupuncture and Chinese herbal medicine seems quite surprising perhaps to the average reader, but not really. Having spent over thirty years translating old and new books and articles on acupuncture and related studies, I am not all that surprised that this has been discovered. What I am surprised by is that it hasn't been discovered much earlier.

Part of the problem is the lack of available source materials. In the early 1990s, I went to my Chinese book supplier in Melbourne, Australia, and gave them a list of Chinese medical titles I copied from a Chinese dictionary and a Chinese medicine encyclopaedia and asked them to get me these books. They were unable to comply. In fact, one of the quite well-known books, the *Pi wei lun* (*The Treatise on the Spleen and Stomach*) I was told hadn't been in print since the early 1970s. Given the lack of primary source materials, I am not that surprised people haven't known about the existence of pre-1949 acupuncture or have not written about this before.

Fortunately, by the late 1990s, things were starting to change. Probably because of emerging interest on the subject matter and because the Chinese people were starting to think along a similar basis, the PRC began publishing a lot of materials, which undoubtedly hadn't seen the light of day for many, many decades.

A lot of the revival of this literature gave me the impetus or start to rediscover what is essentially the missing understanding of TCM. (In fact, when you study *The Treatise on the Spleen and Stomach,* which is now available in China, there are many references to this old, old system).

The only major thing then I will say, to commend more modern doctors of Chinese medicine is regarding the Qing Dynasty (1644–1911), the last dynasty in China. The Qing Dynasty was notable not only for its production of the wen bing classics, which were the result of Westerners interacting with China during this time, but also their assessment and treatment of some more difficult disease conditions. For example, take this Qing herbal prescription to name one (from the *Qing dai ming yi yi an jing hua,* 1981 edition, p.46) *(Qing dynasty medicine document for special care beautiful book)*:

Ren shen   jie geng   wu yao   mu xiang   tian dong

<u>eat with bai jin wan.</u>

The explanation of this prescription (even though it is herbal) is: 'depression injures the heart yang, the yang collapses into yin, become *lin chong.* Emotions and feelings internally injure, similarly becomes yin xu illness . . .' So the Qing Dynasty doctors believed there was more than just heart yang xu (deficiency), but that this could also involve heart yin xu. Obviously, they knew there was a lot more to the zang-fu syndromes than was originally considered.

(The Qing Dynasty, one should note, is also significant concerning the publication of the *Yi zong jin jian* (*Medical and Academic Learning from the Golden Mirror*). This once more was an affirmation of what had gone before and was originally commissioned by the authorities as an attempt to summarise the essentials of Chinese medicine. Once more, we can see a move being made to 'weed through the old'.

Unfortunately, as this book has shown, this attempt was somewhat limited.

In conclusion, both the early thoughts on acupuncture and TCM as well as the thoughts of doctors of the Qing Dynasty are being rediscovered. While the ideas of the first few dynasties are vastly different from today's views on acupuncture, etc., so too are the ideas of the Qing Dynasty in this regard, basically showing that Chinese medicine has not only the advantage of being thousands of years old but can evolve (for the better) if need be. Also, there is no need for the Chinese (communists) to come up with a 'better mousetrap'.

CHAPTER 8

Different Thinking

Part of the reason why pre-1949 acupuncture and TCM have remained hidden for centuries, even thousands of years, is from the lack of adequate source materials—this has already been stated. However, part of the reason for pre-1949 acupuncture, etc., in the first place is 'lateral thinking'. Whereas in the West, people are besotted with 'linear thinking', that is, that which follows on from something else, to illustrate:

Figure 4

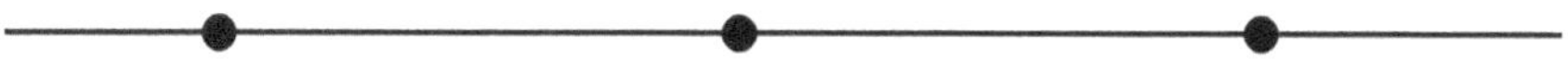

While people have no knowledge of anything being wrong in the first place, we blindly carry on building on what may be incorrect after all. The best example of this is the idea that once existed that the Earth was flat and that the sun revolved around it. This was the cornerstone of the church's thinking for hundreds of years. Later, people like Galileo and Copernicus changed all this. (Likewise, the only advantage of basing Chinese medicine on a Western system is that it simply gives credence to acupuncture and TCM in theory, and when it fails to work in practicality, it may lose its support altogether).

On the other hand, the doctors who originally wrote about acupuncture and TCM used a vastly different form of thinking. They were much more 'lateral thinkers'. In other words, they weren't interested in engaging in conclusions based on past, possibly wrong, assumptions. Instead, they started from a point in space and worked out from there.

And, at times, these 'crystallisations of thoughts' ended up (not intentionally) touching one another.

Figure 5

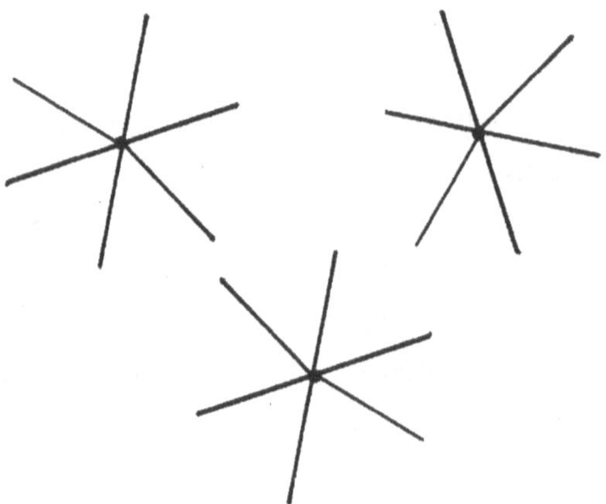

This is actually called 'yuan ci' (original thinking). 'Original thinking is a fundamental characteristic: everything, whether sky, the natural environment, plants, etc., i.e., all things affect each other. It is a very complex concept which cannot be analysed with logic' *(Shen mi de xing xiang)*. This view is not only discussed in Chinese books but also by Western writers, particularly in France.

By comparison, Western thinking is not as 'intellectual' as some people have erroneously complained about, but it is more 'divisional' and 'analytical' as has really been the case. This aids in many of the pitfalls of current modes of thinking and therefore tends to define true traditional Chinese medicine.

CHAPTER 9

Where Do We Go From Here?

First and foremost, do the different schools of thought play a part in pre-1949 acupuncture? The answer is, of course. But as we've said, they may be the result and not the cause of many people's problems. (Included in this is: Shang han, Zang fu, Za bing, and Wen bing, etc.). Hence, they may not be considered by doctors as the sole, independent cause of illnesses and in reality passing concerns.

Secondly, what about the different microsystems? The two types of ear acupuncture, the four or five types of scalp acupuncture, suture acupuncture, and point injection acupuncture, etc.? Are they compatible with pre-1949 acupuncture? Again, yes. The only thing practitioners have to remember is not to reduce the role of pre-1949 acupuncture and not let anything affect its effectiveness.

Thirdly, what about the qi jing ba mai (the eight extraordinary channels)? Because they are an internally connected system (which results in something like reservoirs, as Professor Guan Zun hui has described them) and because they are not affected directly by the year, the season, or the climate, etc., they are not involved in this discussion of pre-1949 acupuncture. In other words, they are a separate system and their symptomatology (or jing jing bing hou) can be taken at face value *(Zhen jiu xue, 1985 p.66,67)*.

Du mai: hands and feet zhu ruan (convulsions), shaking, tension, stroke can't speak, xian illness (epilepsy), dian kuang (manic depressive behaviour), head parts painful and eyes red swelling painful, have tears, legs knees waist back painful, neck hardness, shang han (typhoid?), throat or teeth swelling painful, hands and feet ma (numb), tetanus, self-sweating.

Ren mai: zhi illness (haemorrhoids, piles), diarrhoea, stools like slurry, nue ji (malaria), cough, vomiting blood, urine with blood, teeth painful, throat swelling, urine is not very well, chest wan (gastric cavity) abdomen parts painful, stroke after having a baby, waist painful, dead body retained inside the mother and can't go out, umbilicus and abdomen have a cold feeling, vomiting, hiccups, breasts painful, beng lou, etc.

Chong mai: heart wan painful, chest wan full and stuffy, blocked chest, regurgitation, indigestion, intestines have sounds, stools like slurry, yan ge (cancer of the oesophagus), breathing hurried, ribs distended, umbilicus and abdomen pain, intestinal wind, stools with blood, malaria, retained lochia, after having a baby lost consciousness.

Dai mai: stroke, hands and feet paralysis, limbs painful and numb tense, have fever, head wind painful, neck cheek/jaw swelling, eyes red painful, toothache, throat swelling, dizziness, deafness, skin wind rash (feng zhen) itchy, tendons and mai tense and uncomfortable, legs painful, ribs painful.

Yin qiao mai: throat qi blocked, urine can't finish and dripping, urinary bladder qi painful, intestines have sounds, intestinal wind bleeding out, vomiting, diarrhoea, regurgitation, difficulty in having stools, difficulty in giving birth, loss of consciousness, blockage in the abdomen, diaphragm bad qi, globus hystericus (mei he qi), jaundice (huang dan).

Yang qiao mai: waist and back hardness, big swelling, frightened of wind, self-sweating, headache, storm head wind, head has sweating, eyes red and painful, corner of eye-bone painful, bone joints sour and painful, tense, jue xi (jue adverse), chui you (blue breasts), deafness, nose bleeding, dian xian, swelling of whole body.

Yin wei mai: chest wan full stuffy (pi man) distended, intestines have sounds, diarrhoea, tuo gang (prolapse of anus), fan wei (regurgitation), cancer of the oesophagus, blockage of the abdomen (pi kuai), ribs painful, women's ribs painful, heart painful, chest blockage (jie xiong), shang han, malaria.

Yang wei mai: shang han have a fever, sweating, joints swollen painful, head & nape of neck pain, corner of eyebrow-bone painful, hands and feet hot, numb (fa ma), back hips & tendons bones painful, four limbs are not comfortable, night-sweating, tetanus, knee parts have a cold feeling, heel swelling, eyes red painful.

Fourthly, 'shi dong' and 'suo sheng bing'? This more traditional pre-1949 acupuncture doesn't negate these ideas. In fact, a lot of the symptoms described under the heading of 'triumph' are very much like 'shi dong' and 'suo sheng bing'.

Fifthly and finally, what about the different types of acupuncture? Japanese acupuncture, Korean acupuncture, and Indian acupuncture, to name a few?

When looking at a lot of books and articles on these respective countries' (and also others') massage and acupressure, I am struck by the similarity with Chinese massage etc., so much so that I can name every technique that I see in Chinese. This is not to say, that various countries don't have their own discoveries (which may have flowed through to China) and own nuances but very few people, especially in the West, would really be able to tell these differences from whether they occur on a national level or an individual-practitioner level, regardless of how large the practitioner's school is.

Similarly, and I hate to shock the reader, but there is no difference between Chinese acupuncture and say, Japanese acupuncture. (At the beginning of this book, I was at great pains to show that acupuncture is not just Chinese, that it belongs, from what evidence we do possess, to world history). What we now call Japanese acupuncture (i.e., shallow needling and no retention of needles, etc.) is in actuality, original Chinese acupuncture from the *Nei Jing-Su wen* and before. This all changed with the advent of the *Ling shu* which recommended the deeper insertion of needles and the longer retention of needles in order to better combat deficient and cold diseases (*Zhen jiu xue*, 1985 p.18). (Along the same lines, I was told that today, in China, it is not uncommon to leave needles in for almost an hour when treating cold-deficient stomach ulcers). Obviously, what has happened is that at certain times, when both China and Japan were on better terms and had more 'open-door' policies, more cultural and intellectual exchange went on between the two countries, and so Japanese acupuncture history is more stilted and developed, during certain periods, on its own accord. What we are seeing under the guise of Japanese acupuncture is really very old parts of traditional Chinese acupuncture preserved and perhaps somewhat altered over the course of time and relabelled under the name of either Japanese acupuncture or some particular prefecture's acupuncture. This is also not to say that the Japanese didn't make their own discoveries, like in the case of massage. In fact, when I was in China, the Chinese were quite, and surprisingly, complimentary about Japanese views and developments.

The same can be said regarding many other national forms of acupuncture. No doubt there was some exchange of ideas and interplay between the many Asian nations, but China has remained the centre of acupuncture development for many thousands of years and, despite some evidence to the contrary, was one of its early users, if not necessarily the sole originator, of this system of medicine.

In addition, acupuncture may have changed a lot over thousands of years and not necessarily for the better. As we have seen, the early pre-1949 acupuncture may well had been 'losing ground' since early times, even as far back as *The Pulse Classic* or, at least, some people's subsequent renditions of it. The post-1949 PRC may have made acupuncture and TCM easier to understand and learn yet in trying to codify and standardise them, it may have lost some of its innate abilities as well, as a consequence. Having said that, there is still the matter of the Qing Dynasty and its place in Chinese medicine. Like almost an oasis in a veritable desert of significant ideas, the Qing Dynasty not only had to deal with foreign invasions, from near and far, but in some ways was able to rekindle a lot of what had become oppressed knowledge and understanding.

To go into many of the specifics of pre-1949 acupuncture perhaps would not only do it injustice but would be pretty well impossible to undertake. Not only do acupuncture and Chinese herbal medicine take a long time to learn, but some may never understand it all. This is very different from manufacturing cars on an assembly line or mass educating people as many nations have tried to do in the past. It is different from reading some articles on the internet or discussing things on some website with a hundred others. And yet, this understanding seems to have been around for thousands of years old and new. Is pre-1949 acupuncture simply a legacy of the ancient Chinese people, or is it really a legacy left by all the ancient peoples of the world to all the people of the new world?

LIST OF TERMS

Cun, guan, chi – Inch, bar, and cubit pulses in Western medicine terminology, respectively.

Ming men – 'Life gate'; perhaps equivalent to the adrenal glands in Western medicine.

Tai yang point – Actually not the extra/new acupuncture point, but GB3 in ancient times.

Tan zhong – the chest centre.

Tian di – heaven and earth. The human body is considered a microcosm of nature.

Tian quan – heaven and the 'bubbling spring'. The beginning and the end of a disease process in a year.

Triple heater – The three (burning) spaces around the viscera and the bowels. It has its own channel.

Yin yang – Some people refer to them as 'the feminine' and 'the masculine' in principle. However, suffice to say, they are considered complementary opposites in Oriental philosophy and represent many similar concepts.

Ying, bu ying – 'Suitable' and 'unsuitable'; in other words, re 'ying', something may be 'appropriate' but not necessarily ideal, just expected.

RECOMMENDED READINGS

Huang di nei jing su wen yun qi qi pian jiang jie.

Qing dai ming yi yi an jing hua, 1981 edition *(Qing Dynasty Medicine Document For Special Care Beautiful Book):*

Xue gu zhen ze, 1991

Zhong guo yi xue zhen fa da zhen, 1991

Zhang zhong jing's *shang Han Lun*

Yi zong jin jian (Medical and Academic Learning from the Golden Mirror)

Zhong guo yi xue fa da jin, 1991

Pi wei lun (The Treatise on Spleen and Stomach) by Li Dong yuan

Mai Jing, Wang shu he

Zhen jiu xue, 1985

Shan han jin gui wen bing ming zhu ji cheng

ANDREW MCPHERSON

Andrew McPherson has a bachelor of arts in modern Asian studies from Griffith University and is a government-recognised member of AHPRA. He has been a doctor of Chinese medicine for at least thirty years. He is the president of the Australian National Acupuncturists and Chinese Herbalists Association and has written numerous articles for newspapers, magazines, and books. In addition, he has studied in the People's Republic of China for extended periods. He is a long-term student of Professor Guan Zun hui.

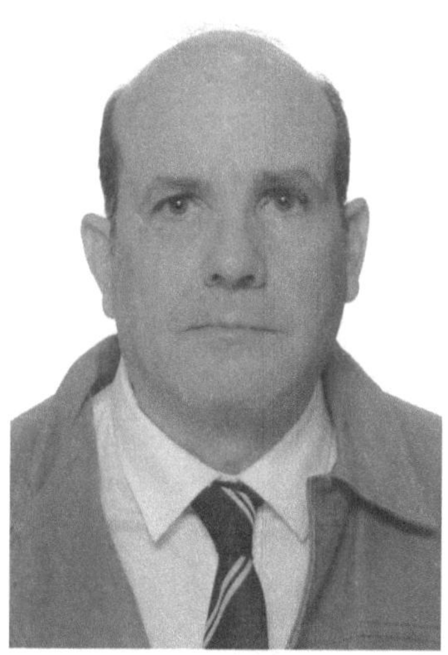

www.ingramcontent.com/pod-product-compliance
Lightning Source LLC
Chambersburg PA
CBHW051419250726